GMO

MW01095128

GMO

How To Avoid Foods That Ruin Your Life - GMO Foods, Organic Food & Food Addiction

Respective authors own all copyrights not held by the publisher.

Legal Notice:
This book is copyright protected. This is only for personal use. You cannot amend, distribute, sell, use, quote or paraphrase any part or the content within this book without the consent of the author or copyright owner. Legal action will be pursued if this is breached.

Disclaimer Notice:
Please note the information contained within this document is for educational and entertainment purposes only. Every attempt has been made to provide accurate, up to date and reliable complete information. No warranties of any kind are expressed or implied. Readers acknowledge that the author is not engaging in the rendering of legal, financial, medical or professional advice.

Table of Contents

Introduction

This book has been written specifically to help you to identify different types of food that aren't genetically enhanced. GMOs were specifically altered to help in the battle against food shortage and malnutrition.

However, the good intentions of the researchers have been shadowed by the profit domineering companies that promote GMOs. Genetics is a broad subject that needs to be handled responsibly.

Alterations done to any organism can be construed as playing God because changes done to the DNA can also alter the way of life of the organism. Consequently these changes will also affect the environment that it inhabits. These are all ripple effects that could ultimately affect humans adversely.

This book contains risk factors of GMO food consumption. This is valuable information that can help in citing for possible effects in the future. These risk factors should be taken seriously because most of the food on the dinner table may very well contain GMOs.

Find out more about GMOs and its effects and be informed on how to avoid these "well intentioned" products that can cause a great deal of trouble in the future.

A Brief History

The appearance of pests and the need for proper nutrition in Third World countries has prompted genetic engineers to pursue altering the genetic makeup of some types of organisms. The purpose of this endeavor is to ensure that any lack of supply in food would be overcome. All of this was done for the good of mankind.

GMO or Genetically Modified Organisms are organisms whose inherent composition has been changed through genetic engineering. Through this process, genetic engineers have more control over the organism's genetic structure than through the usually breeding process.

Genetic engineering has enabled staple crops withstand certain pathogens and herbicides. The process has even ensured that all nutrients will be present for the benefit of nutrition.

The human civilization has been applying their knowledge to food production since the beginning of time.

The development of methods used in improving products goes back to early civilizations. Back then, yeast and malt played a major part in the food development.

Their crude processes were a prelude of man's need for learning new methods in food processing. The invention of the microscope has given man additional arsenal in his quest for knowledge.

The microscope provided a whole new insight on new discoveries which put more fuel into the fire. This lead to more discoveries as to how food is processed and each step is carefully monitored.

Scientists were able see windows of opportunity in improving the properties of certain organisms. Some were even able to alter crops to resists herbicide.

Herbicides are substances that are used to eliminate weeds or other unwanted plant life. There is a question on how this change would affect the environment as well as the people consuming the product.

Nowadays, genetic engineers are busy in finding different ways to develop and improve a variety of organisms. The processes whereby they alter the genetic materials of these organisms are in open debate. There are several controversies that surround the creation and consumption of GMO food. A lot of people are concerned of the effects of GMO food to the health of consumers. There are also questions on how the GMO can be regulated.

In Europe, the labeling of products containing GMO ingredients is required by the law. However, in the US and Canada it is at the discretion of the manufacturer if they are going to add that information in their labels.

There is an ongoing fight to ensure that all manufacturers have to properly label their products for the good of the consumers.

The Risks Involved

GMOs can provide a lot of solutions to society's problems with regard to lack of food, development of vaccines, malnutrition, etc. However no matter how good the intentions of these researchers and genetic engineers were or are, there's still a human ethical issues at hand.

People feel that there is a lack in proper testing of the foodstuffs. There might be possible negative effects that these new improved organisms bring into ecosystems and to mankind in general.

Religious organizations, environmental groups and civic groups have been voicing their concerns of the adverse effects of the creation of GMOs in the environment.

These groups expressed different issues that seem to follow the wake of GMOs infamy. The groups feel that the inherent characteristics of some crops to resist the effect of herbicide and some pests, they feel that this characteristic would ultimately affect the other insects and plant life that doesn't harm the crops.

Since these new crops have new capabilities that will be introduced to an ecosystem it's important to know what they are.

The other organisms within that ecosystem may react differently to a newcomer. There might be an instance where an organism may lose their niche and cease to exist. The cross-pollination of plants might also transfer the ability to resist herbicides to the weeds which of course is unwanted.

The target organism will have a means to protect itself and this may cause weeds to outgrow the crop population. An enhanced weed population would be able to successfully compete with the rest of the plants in the ecosystem.

This could cause a great imbalance and may be the cause of a loss of certain species that rely on that environment. Since there are enhanced crops that are altered to contain their own pesticides, these may in turn enable the insects to be resistant to pesticides.

There are certain risks to humans that these groups are concerned about. There are people who are allergic to certain types of food like nuts. If certain properties of nuts were to be transferred to another crop, this may cause another allergen to develop.

There are a lot of "what if's" that could happen when it comes to genetics. The question of the effect of GMOs on humans is still a question being asked until today. All research has been inconclusive and there is certain information going around that arouses the growing panic of the public against these enhanced products.

All the research that is being conducted will cost a lot of money. This means that there should be a return on investment for the people who have given substantial funds for the research to be successful.

If there are huge amounts of funds used on the research, the purpose of providing a sustainable harvest to the farmers and to people in Third World countries through the research would be for naught.

Companies who funded the research would still want to get the maximum profit from the investment.

Why Choose a GMO Free Diet?

The growing panic of parents about the long term effects of GMO foods has made them clamor for ways to avoid these rampant products and still be able to get all the nutritional values from GMO free foods.

But why do we need to pursue an all-natural diet? What does the body get from it?

Studies show that combining traits from other organisms to enhance properties of another plant may cause allergens to be created. So, even if a certain product has no allergens originally, in the end, it may develop new allergens that can cause long term illnesses. The fact is, it's an unknown quantity.

These types of allergens may prolong conditions for patients with chronic illness. Physicians strongly suggest that patients avoid GMO foods and stick to non-GMOs or ideally organic products.

This process hastens recovery and improves the general condition of the patient health wise.

It seems that the natural components of Non-GMO products aid the patient's recovery process.

There has been significant study showing the adverse effect of GMO products on the body with long term use. Among these is the increase in the infertility rate, aging, interruption in the proper insulin regulation, changes in the major body organs, problems in the immune system and gastrointestinal problems.

These are pretty serious complications that can further develop with continued consumption of GMO food. Parents are concerned about the welfare and health of their children.

It is important to ensure that the food provides proper nutrition and won't leave any negative after effects. There are studies showing how laboratory mice that were fed by GMO soy had an increase in infant death when compared with those that were fed with natural soy.

Even the male rats' organs were changed due the introduction of GMO food. Their testicles turned blue after regular feeding. There are even accounts of increased death rates in livestock and poultry all over the world.

Through continued consumption, people have unwittingly become guinea pigs due to the lack of intensive testing on GMOs.

On the other hand, all natural products have been fulfilling mankind's needs for sustenance and nutrition. Although there have been real problems when it comes to adequate supply due to natural problems like changes in weather and pests, it is still the best source of food, hands down. It is also the safest source of nutrition to date.

Organic farming is the most earth-friendly way of producing food. It lessens soil erosion. This means there would be less damage to property and human life when there are natural disasters. It can also lessen the presence of pesticides in the soil.

Organic farming doesn't use pesticides which is good for pregnant women because pesticides can even reach the unborn child. This also contributes to infertility problems and birth defects. Organic products don't have these problems to contend with because they are grown without the use of chemicals.

It's Time To Go
Organic

The change from regular food to organic products can be a real pain in the wallet. Organic food doesn't come cheap. However, the benefit that it can provide is priceless to your body.

There are certain ways to get organic food at a discount like going to food fairs or buying it when it is in season. It is quite hard to get organic food all year round if the price is a hindrance.

The best way to get organic food all the time would be to grow it yourself. It can be a daunting task for those who have never grown anything. Growing organic food means that pesticides and synthetic fertilizers will not be used ever. It is better to start small, like growing two plants first for easier management.

The first thing to consider in organic farming is the condition of the soil. Since synthetic fertilizers should be out of the picture it is better to use humus, an organic component used to help soil hold water and nutrients. Humus is mixed with dried leaves, and manure.

This would help condition the soil as opposed to synthetic fertilizers which can harm the good bacteria and worms in the soil. Make sure that the compost is turned regularly and add dried leaves or sawdust if in case it smells.

This would minimize the smell especially if the space is limited. Next choose the best type of plant to grow. It is better to choose the ones that can easily adapt to its environment. Check with local growers on which plants are the best to grow each season.

Seedlings can be another option. These can be purchased from farmer's market. Ask which seedlings are native to the area. These are the ones that can easily adapt to the soil and the climate. For gardens that have limited spaces it is better to plant tomatoes, pole beans, zucchini and snow peas.

These are plants that continuously branch out and bear fruit until winter.

Caring for the plants will be the activity that will be needed to be done most of the time. It is better to water the plants in the morning and should be focused on the roots.

Even if the space is small there is still a possibility that weeds can grow with the plants. Pulling weeds is a good form of exercise. But adding mulch to the soil can minimize the presence of weeds. Mulch is a material that is placed on the top of the soil to insulate it and suppress weeds.

Natural material like leaves, bark of trees and compost are the best kind of mulch. When it decomposes, it will enrich the soil which is better for the plants. The presence of pests can be an indication that the plant has a deeper problem. Make sure that the garden is getting enough light, moisture and nutrients.

Natural predators like lizards, frogs and birds can also help the garden get rid of harmful pests. If there are sick plants in the garden it is a good practice to remove the whole plant and rake the soil. Anything that is left from the sick plant can also affect the healthier plants around it.

It takes a lot of time and effort to maintain a garden but the fruits of the labor can be very sweet indeed. For newbies, it is better to start a small garden and then expand once you gain more experience.

Tips and Tricks

The clamor for a GMO free diet has been going around for the past years. People have become more aware of the things that they put on the dinner table. The ever present danger of GMO consumption has become a constant nightmare for the parents today.

A lot of individuals are very conscious about the kinds of food that they eat. They are very conscious of the things they put into their bodies. For those who are nervous about buying GMO foods there are certain guidelines that can be followed.

The most common crops that have been genetically altered are soy, corn, canola and cotton. The seeds of these crops are herbicide resistant and a contract is signed by the farmer to buy herbicide from the company who sold the seed. These seeds are altered for maximum harvest. Cattle is affected indirectly by GMO the food that they eat. One way to ensure that GMO food is avoided is by buying organic food.

There is a strict monitoring of organic farming by the USDA. No organic seeds are used because of the strict compliance. Try to look for non-GMO labels in products. Sometimes these are labeled as "produced without genetically modified ingredients." Check the most common ingredients that are used to see if they are GMO.

It is better to avoid the crops that are usually used as GMO. As previously stated corn, soy, canola and cotton are products that are at risk when it comes to GMO.

Try to use alternative crops and eat more fruits and vegetables. These are mostly organic crops which are better for overall health.

Processed foods are more than likely to have been produced by using GMO food. Even if the contents are checked there is still a big possibility that some or most of the ingredients are genetically modified.

Artificial sweetener called aspartame is also a risk because it is created through the use of GM microorganisms. Artificial sweeteners are mostly used for losing weight. But in this case there are certain controversies that cannot be avoided.

There are studies that show that this can cause cancer, birth defects, vision problems, diabetes and can a hindrance in losing weight. Poultry raised in the range is a better choice for meat.

These are fed with organic feeds. Most dressed chickens are very likely fed with GMO corns. For beef it is better to check if they are 100% grass-fed. It is important to remain vigilant in ensuring that all the food that is placed on your table a dinner is tamper proof.

Even if the intentions of GMO producers are spotless, there are still a lot of unknown factors that play a role as a result of introducing these types of food into the system.

It is important to ensure that this will not happen in the future. There are certain kinds of risks that are not worth the good that they can provide. The few dollars that can be saved by buying cheap products can cause huge amounts of money in health care in the future.

Finding GMO Free Food

Not everyone has the capacity and the space to create an organic garden. Most people rely on shopping to get their supply of food. These are the ones that are too busy or have too little space for the garden. Shopping for organic or Non-GMO food can be really tiresome.

It is better to check the brands of certain foods online to see if they belong to Non-GMO products. There are shopping lists for Non-GMO products that can be referred to before going on a shopping trip.

Buying organic products on the market is also another means of ensuring that the food being purchased is all natural. It is better to buy products that are in season because these are the ones that are cheaper. Going to farmer's markets can also be another option.

Most local farmers sell non-GMO produce. There are also certain manufacturers that don't use GMO food in their products. Since there are no laws on labeling yet, some manufacturer have opted to add "Non-GMO" to their labels.

Supermarkets also have put numbers on a label for fruits and vegetables. This can help shoppers in identifying which are Non-GMO products. If it's a four digit number then the product is organic. If it starts with a 9 and is a five digit number it's a GMO product. If the product starts with an 8 and is a five digit number then it's a Non-GMO product.

There are certain mobile applications that also can help in identifying which brands are Non-GMO.

Application developers have noted the needs of shoppers to find naturally produced food. It takes a lot of time and effort to go around the market just to find the right products.

The Non-GMO Project is an iPhone app that can show the list of brands that continue to uphold the production of all natural food. The application can be used to search through brand lists, keywords and products.

It can be a difficult task to find Non-GMO products; it's a good thing that there are ways to lessen the time and effort of finding them.

Conclusion

I hope that I was able to help you and that this book was able to give you more information on GMO foods. The problem that most people have is because of the Government's stance on labeling which would be a lot easier for people if the European stance was adopted, where clear marking shows which foods contain GMO products.

The safest bet is always going to be to produce your own foods or to buy from a Farmer's Market because you know what you are getting. As you can see from the book, we are being used as guinea pigs and if the results on rats and mice are anything to go by, this is worrying.

If in doubt, try to stick to brands that you know do not use GMO products and you can research this much more easily these days. The Free Thought project has a list of 400 companies that do not use GMO products and this may be a helpful clue to you as to which companies are safe to trust. This list is found at the link below and if you cannot link directly, simply paste it into your browser.

http://thefreethoughtproject.com/400-companies-gmos-products/

Be safe and know what you and your family are eating.

Conclusion

Just one more thing: *Can I ask you one last question?*

Well, how do you feel? Do you feel enthusiastic about what you've learned, overwhelmed or simply indifferent? I hope you feel at least something.

If so, share it with other readers!

Enter the following URL

http://amzn.to/1LKSC3d

or simply visit the product page, scroll down and click on this following button.

Share your thoughts with other customers

Write a customer review

Even if it's just 1 sentence, it would make me super happy! Reviews like yours can truly make the difference between a book selling or not – other readers get an idea of what to expect.

NOTE: Share your honest feedback whether it's positive or negative! If you didn't like this book, tell us why! We want to know, so we can improve the quality. That's why feedback/reviews are invaluable.

The following pages are for taking notes.